2014 Version
Copyright © Arie Bergs
All rights reserved
ISBN 10: 1511886951
ISBN 13: 9781511886956
Translated from "OORSUIZEN – 100 remedies"

.

In advance

Because it is my primary intention to provide a list of remedies for tinnitus in this book, I will never delve into the history of therapies described or the manufacturers or origins of certain remedies. There has been no effort made to advertise any product here. In addition, I will not give general description of hearing, the brain or the body in general within this book. Libraries are full of books on the science of medicine and how the human body functions. Because I myself am a tinnitus patient, and a handbook with 100 remedies for tinnitus has not yet existed anywhere in the world, in writing this, I hope to help a few fellow tinnitus sufferers.

.

Contents

.

Introduction

I know people with intense tinnitus, who remain passive toward tinnitus because their doctor told them no cure exists and their tinnitus will never be reduced. As long as there is no "magical" remedy that cures tinnitus, in the way there is aspirin for migraines, these people will do nothing.

On the other hand, there are people like you and me, who will read this book. People who grab the bull by the horns. People who take initiative and who would give anything to reduce their tinnitus. People who will undoubtedly find one or more solutions in this book that will benefit them. People who are willing to change their lifestyle. It is well-known that there is no magic cure for tinnitus. Still, there are people who are helped in whole or in part by some sort of remedy every day.

The chiropractor, the osteopath and physiotherapist can help. The GP and the ENT doctor rely mostly on traditional medicine and prescribing traditional pharmaceuticals. Acupuncture, homeopathy, healthy eating, sport and exercise supplements, tai-chi and foot reflexology also provide help.

Like me, many people have had to deal with tinnitus for a long time. At any given moment, the internet, libraries, lectures, bookstores and magazines are being scoured for a way to make this whistling, rustling, buzzing, roaring go away. Eventually you won't be able to see the forest from the trees and you'll have already paid a fortune for therapies, potions, pills and devices.

This is why I've written this book, *Tinnitus- 100 Remedies,* in which I attempt to put everything in a nutshell. The number 100 can be thought of as a rather arbitrary number in this context. Surely there are 100 remedies. Homeopathy alone discusses at least 30 ways to reduce tinnitus. Medicinal herbs are abundant and the number of tinctures against tinnitus seems unlimited.

Weekly, if not daily, the pharmaceutical industry puts a product on the market that would also be capable of suppressing tinnitus. Numerous therapies already exist, and as far as healthy eating is concerned, there are hundreds of types of food. So, as you can see, I could easily have used the number 99, 101 or 157.

.

1   Tinnitus & Hyperacusis

There is no more sensitive detecting instrument than the human body.

1.1   Tinnitus

Tinnitus, a technical term for ringing in the ears, is a disorder of the acoustic system which is accompanied by hearing sounds from hissing, whistling, buzzing, humming, alternating beeps to the sound of a jet. The name tinnitus comes from the Latin *Tinnitus Aurium,* or *tinnire,* which means ringing. Tinnitus is not exclusive to this day and age. In 1650 BC, the Egyptians were already talking about a "buzzing in the ear."

Tinnitus is completely unpredictable and can affect anyone.

Famous people who have or have had tinnitus include: Phil Collins, Eric Clapton, Sting, Bono, Cher, Neil Young, Barbra Streisand, Ronald Reagan, Maarten Luther, Charles Darwin, Jean-Jacques Rousseau, Jeanne d'Arc, Ludwig Von Beethoven, Vincent van Gogh, and the list goes on.

Everyone has suffered briefly from tinnitus that disappears as suddenly as it occurs. When this acute tinnitus exists for more than four to six months, it is then termed chronic tinnitus.

Vigorous tinnitus in one ear is torture and violent tinnitus in both ears is a living nightmare. The tinnitus may occasionally be so strong that one can not sleep. After some time, tinnitus can lead to concentration problems. In addition, intense tinnitus is accompanied by feelings of helplessness and depression. As a result, quality of life can be severely compromised. Tinnitus this severe becomes so disruptive that people living with the condition become incapable of normally participating in everyday life.

Overactivity in the auditory part of the brain results in signals continuing to be sent when sound is no longer present. This is referred to as phantom sound. The source of tinnitus remains unknown. In 30% of the cases, an exact cause, such as noise, can be established. In all other cases, identifying a cause essentially becomes a guessing game. Initially, the doctor will look for blood flow disorders.

According to statistics, the number of people with tinnitus increases linearly (especially in industrialized countries). Today, more than 10% of the population suffers from tinnitus. That's one million Belgians, 1.5 million Dutchmen, 7 million Frenchmen and about 50 million Americans. This is largely due to the frequent visits to festivals, the use of earphones for MP3 players, the overuse of medication, drugs, alcohol and especially the stress and excitement in the modern world. Now is the time to educate people and do something about it.

1.2   Hyperacusis

Hyperacusis, from a Greek word meaning "too much hearing" is a hypersensitivity to sound that causes someone to develop earaches in reaction to everyday sounds. The cause remains unknown. Everyday sounds that are problematic include chirping birds, crying children, doorbells, ringing telephones, vacuum cleaners, hair dryers, cutlery scratching a plate or stirring with a spoon, and more. Voices sound shrill. Conversations in a group are out of the question and walking on a hardwood floor with high heels causes headaches. People with hyperacusis cannot tolerate normal ambient noise. In today's society in particular, hyperacusis is an unmitigated disaster.

Approximately 30% of tinnitus patients also appear to suffer from hyperacusis. Someone with hyperacusis has no choice but to change his or her habits and pursuits or even completely cast them to the side.

Tinnitus and hyperacusis are especially difficult obstacles to overcome as science still cannot provide a proper explanation of their cause with certainty.

1.3   Possible causes

Precisely how tinnitus arises remains unknown to this day. There is an abundant amount of possible causes; the primary factor is noise, followed by stress, illness and medication. I will not talk about the functioning of our hearing, the sophisticated physiological process, or the conversion of mechanical noise to electronic sound that occurs through our nervous system in this book. Anyone with tinnitus who reads this book has already searched the internet and has read about what tinnitus actually is and how hearing works repeatedly. It comes down to the fact that there is an imbalance of electrical charges between our ears and our brain. Still, below I will give a small list of possible causes. You might find something that directly relates to the remedies mentioned further in this book. A clue can be the start to the solution.

- *Very loud noises* are considered the primary cause of tinnitus. A visit to a nightclub or festival may cause acute hearing loss after as little as 10 minutes. Almost 15% of young people suffer from some form of this, with permanent hearing damage as a result. Listening to music on an mp3 player or iphone through earbuds, for example, at a high volume can be devastating and may result in permanent hearing damage.

- *Hearing loss due to aging:* The risk of developing tinnitus increases with age, particularly after age 50. (In the medical word, this is referred to as presbycusis).

- *Emotional stress*: Stress, fatigue, burnout, depression, panic, anxiety and post-traumatic disorders all cause tinnitus.

- *Trauma*: This includes skull fractures, whiplash or barotrauma.

- *Injuries to the eardrum or a skull injury*.

- *Medication*: Many drugs contain ototoxic substances, including the following medication in particular:

- Diuretics: diuretic agents.
- Aspirin-containing painkillers such as paracetamol and ibuprofen.
- Quinine and chloroquine: for tinnitus after a vacation in the tropics.
- Indometacine: against rheumatic diseases.
- Propranolol : a beta-blocker for heart arrhythmia and hypertension.
- Carbamazepine: for epilepsy and certain neurological disorders.
- Calcium channel blockers
- Aminoglycoside: antibiotics.
- Antihistaminica
- Statinen
- Indomethacin: for pain conditions in the musculoskeletal system.
- Diclofenac: for pain and anti-inflammatory.
- Cisplatina: anti-cancer.
- Anti-malaria medication
- Blood sugar and blood fat lowering medication.
- Aspirin and related nonsteroidal species such as benoxaprofen, feprazone, ibuprofen, carprofen, diclofenac, fenoprofen, and so on. Aspirin has been considered harmless for a long time. Still, chemical composition, initially derived from the willow bark, if overused can have disastrous effect on the circulation, tinnitus, stomach bleeding and rashes from bleeding skin.

- **Sudden deafness**: usually unilateral hearing loss. The cause of this is virtually unknown.

- **High blood pressure, diabetes and atherosclerosis:** falls under the heading of "circulatory disorders" because blood pressure that is either too low or too high can cause tinnitus.

- **Alzheimer's Disease**

- **Otitis Media:** particularly pulsating tinnitus due to a defect in the eardrum.

- **Lyme disease:** transmitted by ticks.

- **Meniere's disease:** accompanied by vertigo, nausea and vomiting.

- **A wax plug**

- **Muscular causes** can occur in the muscles of the Eustachian tube, in the palate muscles or possibly in the muscles of the inner ear, which connect the ossicles.

- **Acoustic neuroma**: a sporadic, benign tumor on the auditory nerve.

- **Otosclerosis**: involves abnormal bone growth in the middle ear. Usually indicates a dip in hearing at 2000 Hz.

- **Gout**

- **Kidney and thyroid ailments**

- **Vitamin deficiency:** such as too little B6 and B12.

- **Cervical spine syndrome**: changes in the cervical spine.

- **Temporomandibular joint:** abrasion in the jaw joint or spasms of the masseter, deep jaw muscles, lateral and medial pterygoid.

- **Teeth:** inflammation of the teeth, ill-adapted dental prosthesis, amalgam fillings, bad teeth particularly in the upper jaw.

- **Allergies:** When the immune system is overloaded, an inactive allergy comes to the surface. Food allergy is especially relevant here. Whole grains, shellfish and eggs are the primary stimulators.

- **Virus infection:** Examples include syphilis, borreliosis, and HIV infection.

- **The pill:** in rare cases.

- **Chronic sinuses**

- **Lack of minerals** such as magnesium and zinc.

- **High hemoglobin levels** that compromise circulation.

- **Hearing loss:** High tone hearing loss usually occurs during old age, loss of mid tones is usually hereditary, and loss of bass tones points to stress. A complete hearing loss of 60 dB usually indicates a complete loss of the outer hair cells in the inner ear.

- **Flight:** when one has a cold during flight, there a change of pressure in the middle of the ear. A traction on the eardrum occurs and fluid retention can cause pain, ringing, hearing loss and possibly a perforation of the eardrum. Treat nose, throat and ear infections before departure.

- **Anaesthetic:** especially during an epidural. With strong decreases in blood pressure, blood flow to the ear may be so greatly reduce that hearing damage results.

- **Disruption in the hormonal system**

- **Brain injury or whiplash**

- **Electromagnetic radiation**

- **Pregnancy**

- **Damage to the capillaries in the inner ear**

- **Iron deficiency**

- **A weak immune system**

- **Rock climbing at high altitude**

- **Scuba diving**

- **Cancer medication:** bromocriptine, cisplatin, vincristine, bleomycin, vinblastine, carboplatin and more.

- **Injectors or solvents:** trichloorethyleen, methyl chloride, styrene, toluol and more

- **Metabolic disorders:** gout, lipid metabolism, kidney and thyroid ailments.

- Additional causes include acoustic neurinoma, ear surgery, Von Hippel-Lindau's disease, swimmers ear and more.

As you can see, it is not surprising that instances of tinnitus are on the rise, and so long as no magical remedy exists, the probability that this will change is quite small. In 40% of cases, the cause of tinnitus cannot be identified.

In the following chapters, I pull out all the stops. All possible treatments and remedies are listed, in no particular order. We'll cover blood thinners to a mustard foot bath; from the squatters (chiropractors) to the sauna. We'll go from masking products to ear candling and from powerful medication to highly diluted homeopathy.

2 Traditional Medicine

Here, I will discuss mainstream medical practices in conjunction with conventional medicine and surgery. Of course, when you're not feeling well, you make an appointment and tell the doctor the whole story. I personally think the doctor should give you confidence. If you don't click with a doctor right away, then I advise you to go look for another one. You are a patient, you pay for the service, and you can decide whether that services is good or bad. Let yourself be treated as a person instead of a number. After all, it is all about your health. Your tinnitus is measured in terms of frequency and loudness. All necessary tests are done to exclude disease and causal factors. Finally, a diagnosis is made.

2.1 Medication

Especially in the early stages of tinnitus the domestic and ENT doctor prescribe antidepressants, tranquilizers and certain mild beta-blockers. Some examples are:

- *Pamelor:* contains nortriptyline and is an antidepressant.

- *Elavil:* contains amitriptyline and is also an antidepressant.

- Xanax: contains alprazolam as a sedative.

- Niravam: also contains alprazolam.

- Rivotril: a classic muscle relaxant.

- Inderal: contains propranolol as a light beta-blocker. Non-selective beta blockers are medicines that slow and maintain the heart rate and lower blood pressure. Inderal is primarily used as a preventive treatment for migraines.

- Seresta: contains oxazepam as a stress-reduction measure. It is a derivative of the family of benzodiazepines and is a tranquilizer.

- Tranxene: contains clorazepate and relieves stress. It's a hypnotic, sedative and anxiolytic. Basically it is a tranquilizer with a long-lasting effect.

- Mogadon: contains nitrazepam. It is a derivative of the group of the benzodiazepines. An effective hypnotic with a long-lasting effect with a risk of cumulative effects, particularly among elderly people.

- Normison: contains temazepam.

- Loramet: contains lormetazepam.

- Temesta: contains lorazepam. An effective sedative with a medium duration.

- Valium: contains diazepam. Has a long-term calming effect but also a relaxing effect on the striated muscles of the body.

- Seroxat: contains paroxetine as an antidepressant.

- Fevarin: contains fluvoxamine as an antidepressant.

- Stilnoct: contains zolpidem as hypnotics.

- Zoloft: contains sertraline to treat depression.

- Paxil: contains paroxetine to treat depression.

- Tegretol: contains carbamazepine for epilepsy and severe nerve pain. This drug has significant side effects.

- Carbimal: also contains carbamazepine.

- Adalat: contains nifedipine as an antihypertensive. Used in some cases of hypertension and may also cause an acceleration of the heart rhythm.

- Xylocaïne: contains lidocaine as a short anesthetic.

- Xylocard: also contains lidocaine as a short anesthetic.

- Campral: medications to treat alcoholism.

- Baclofen: muscle relaxant for migraine attacks.

- Klonopin: consists of clonazepam as sleep aid.

- The list goes on.

In terms of antidepressants, Zoloft, Fevarin and Seroxat are preferred because they inhibit serotonin reuptake. They do not cure tinnitus but ensure that the impact of tinnitus is reduced in terms of mood improvement.

I would not recommend using medications such as Anafranil, Nortrillen, Trypzitol and Sarotex as these are tricyclic antidepressants which are known to not only aggravate existing cases of tinnitus, but also cause new ones.

The disadvantage of antidepressants is that they usually cause a number of side effects such as: decreased appetite, anxiety, nervousness, nausea, diarrhea, agitation, sexual dysfunction and headaches. Most disorders resolve after familiarization with the medication. For a proper effect of antidepressants a use of at least six weeks is required.

For anxiety disorders, Temesta, Seresta, Xanax and Valium are primarily prescribed.

Furthermore, hypnotics like Stilnoct, Loramet, Seresta, Normison and Mogadon may be prescribed for short-term use.

Of course, the medicine cabinet can be further expanded. In any case, consult with your physician is necessary.

Many doctors treat tinnitus directly as a blood circulation disorder and prescribe a blood thinner to allow more oxygen and nutrients to flow through small blood vessels. This not only improves blood flow in the ear, but also does so in other parts of the body.

In fact, there are very few types of medication that target the ear specifically. This also applies to other drugs that are prescribed and which could possibly influence hearing. Often the number of side effects a medication has, can become a deciding factor for whether or not to use them.

Following the test with blood thinners, the doctor will pass to other medications, such as:

- Lidocaïne: a local anesthetic used to control heart rhythm. It can be administered intravenously for a limited period to suppress tinnitus. Usually used in the hospital.

- Anticonvulsants: medication used as a treatment for epilepsy (such as Tegretol made of carbamazepine), as well as for withdrawal symptoms from alcohol and drugs.

- Antiarrhythmic: reduction in the transmission of stimuli through the cell membrane of nerve cells (usually tocaïne sold as xylotocan). Strong stuff that is tolerated by few.

- Antidepressants and tranquilizers: to treat depression, restlessness and dejection. Pay attention here to addiction.

- Glutamate: an IV neurotransmitter that stimulates impulses in the neural pathways. It could suppress pathological spontaneous activity in the auditory pathway. The effectiveness of this has not yet proven.

- Calcium-antagonists: combats coronary heart disease and high blood pressure (eg. flunarizine prescribed as Sibelium, nimodipine prescribed as Nimotop). Calcium channel blockers normalize any wrong influx of calcium.

- Cortisone: (such as Medrol)

- Cinnarizine and Dogmatil (contains sulpiride): combat dizziness.

- Anticonvulsants: only used for severe forms of tinnitus, or after other treatments failed.

Warning: There are hundreds of drugs that cause tinnitus, especially after prolonged use. It will always, and I mean always, be important to read the leaflet. The leaflet is always available, and it's there for a reason.

If a type of medication does not bring you solace after a few months, it no longer makes sense to continue taking it.

2.2 IV Therapy

In some countries, it has been customary to use an IV treatment for cases of acute tinnitus for decades. The main ingredients of such an IV are an anti-inflammatory (prednisolone) and blood thinner (pentoxifylline) that enable better blood flow through the tiny blood vessels in the hearing organ. This treatment should be carried out as soon as possible after the onset of tinnitus. The chance of improvement can be as high as 80%. By improvement, I mean the disappearance of tinnitus or remission. At a later stage, this IV treatment no longer makes sense.

2.3   Surgical operations

Though a last resort, in rare case surgery is the most appropriate treatment. Examples of these rare cases include those where vascular anomalies and an acoustic-neuroma (tumor) are examples. Other cases include the following:

2.3.1   Cortical implant

In this treatment, an electrode is implanted under the skull. This delivers electric shocks to the overactive parts of the brain that are involved in the development of tinnitus, suppressing overactivity and thereby causing tinnitus to become less severe or disappear. Such surgery is currently only accessible to people with very severe tinnitus that can not be treated by any other method and seems to be especially effective if the tinnitus has not existed for a long time.

2.3.2   Jaw surgery

For this you need to see a stomatologist and a dental surgeon.

2.3.3   Cutting the auditory nerve

This surgery is used increasingly less and less as it comes with only a 50% chance of success. This results in a deaf ear without tinnitus or a deaf ear with the same, or possibly worse, tinnitus.

2.3.4   An orthopedic surgeon

An orthopedic surgeon can help if there is any damage to the spine. In particular, the neck portion of the spine may be blocked. In addition, cramped neck and shoulder muscles and/or incorrect positions of the vertebrae be responsible for tinnitus. Of course an x-ray is necessary in this case.

2.3.5   The dentist

Proper maintenance of your teeth, and especially having a bad wisdom tooth removed, may be a solution for your tinnitus. In addition, amalgam fillings in your teeth should be avoided. The mercury therein is pure poison for your nerve cells and organs.

Costen's syndrome

People with Costen's syndrome experience problems with the temporomandibular joint (TMJ) and/or muscles that run along the TMJ. Problems include pain when opening the mouth, cracking or clicking noises when chewing, and blocking or bad closing of the jaw joint.
Possible causes include teeth grinding during sleep, wear and tear osteoarthritis, ill-fitting dentures, detrimental habits like nail biting, poor posture, and muscle tension from stress, including in the head and neck muscles.

3 Body-therapies

In this section, I address our body's structures and systems, including the circulatory system, the lymphatic system, bones and joints.

3.1 Chiropractic care

The name chiropractic is derived from the Greek words cheir (hand) and praxis (action). Therefore, chiropractors' examinations and treatment methods primarily involve the hands. First, a chiropractor will conduct a manual search for changes, malfunctions or erroneous positions of the joints, including the spinal column in particular. The cervical spine comes first, especially for the treatment of tinnitus. Still, providing the chiropractor with a recent x-ray may prove to be useful.

When being treated by a chiropractor, blockages of the joints between the spine are removed and the spine is properly aligned. The corresponding muscles are also discussed.

3.2 Osteopathy

The name osteopathy is derived from the Greek osteon (bone) and pathos (disease). According to the osteopath, the musculoskeletal system plays an important role in the maintenance of homeostasis. Homeostasis is the state of equilibrium in the human body. From a holistic point of view, all parts in our body depend on each other and the whole is mainly influenced by the environment and emotions. Our body is self-regulating and able to heal itself, but if its state of equilibrium is put out of balance as a result of stress, pollution, poor diet or too little rest, diseases arise. In the case of tinnitus, the osteopath will focus on cranial osteopathy.

The tinnitus patient lies in a relaxed position while the osteopath gently manipulates the neck and skull. Through small, gentle manipulative techniques, muscles are normalized. This applies to both relaxed and tense muscles. A cranial osteopath also restores the speed of the cranial rhythmic impulses in the brain and spinal fluid. In addition, this treatment stimulates the lymphatic drainage, as well as the circulation in the brains and head.

3.3 Massage

The word massage is derived from the Greek word *masso*, meaning "kneading." A therapeutic massage, or Swedish massage, is aimed at modifying the soft tissues of the body, such as the skin, muscles, tendons and ligaments. A proper massage has a physiological and a psychological effect. The various manipulations affect not only the skin and the muscles, but also the veins, the lymphatic system, nerves and occasionally the organs. Moreover, a massage has a relaxing effect on the psyche.

In the case of tinnitus, the blood flow, the circulation of the lymph, and the muscles of the neck and the shoulder are stimulated. Particularly for people with tinnitus, massage should always be a pleasant experience, especially for the cervical spine. However, massages that are too powerful can actually have negative effects and may even worsen tinnitus.

Outside of the three aforementioned therapies, there are many body therapies that play an important role physically, as well as psychologically and emotionally. Most therapies I'll name below may be effective for tinnitus, provided you approach a reliable and qualified therapist.

- **Craniosacral therapy** is derived from cranial osteopathy and attaches more importance to the soft tissues in the brains and spinal cord than the bones themselves. The very light craniosacral technique is more esoteric and focuses on loosening the psyche and the physique.

- **The Feldenkrais Method** may be useful in enhancing self-consciousness and reducing stress. The Feldenkrais Method involves a series of easy, fluid movements that mimic everyday postures in order to reprogram the brain. Emphasis is put on re-educating the neuromuscular pathways, rather than simply the muscles.

- **The Alexander Technique** is also effective in reducing stress and resembles much of the Feldenkrais Method. The Alexander Technique works by promoting good breathing, as breathing is influenced by interaction between our head, neck and back.

- **Connective Tissue Massage** is based on the relationship between subcutaneous connective tissues and the corresponding organs, muscles and blood vessels.

- **Dô-in** is largely similar to acupuncture and acupressure. (See below).

- **Lymphatic drainage** involves a massage of the lymphatic system that improves circulation as a result of breathing and muscle movement. This method is particularly useful for people with a hematogenous constitution.

- **Meridian Massage** is no more than a combination of acupuncture and connective tissue massage.

4 Energy therapies

4.1 Acupuncture

Acupuncture is part of traditional Chinese medicine. The name comes from *acus* ("needle") and *punctura* ("stitch"). Needles are used to prick the body on specific acupuncture points that correspond to the meridian system. Because an acupuncture needle is very thin and has a rounded top, puncturing is not normally painful, and chances of bleeding are virtually zero. The meridian system consists of twelve main meridians (energy pathways) and two extra meridians, which together comprise approximately 1,000 acupuncture points. Of these, 361 classical acupuncture points are principally important in terms of their location, name, features and display.

Acupuncture and the meridian systems have been around for thousands of years, whereas mainstream medicine has been around for 150 years. Isn't that something to think about?

Tip: Always go to a licensed acupuncturist. And I do not mean just any therapist with an acupuncture diploma. I mean someone who has studied in China; an acupuncturist who controls the art of traditional medicine. Someone who understands structure and agreements on Yin and Yang. Someone who has an understanding of the five elements of fire, water, earth, wood and metal. I have gone to several acupuncturists and I've found them a bit amateuristic. Most of them just stab around hoping to see improvement. It is not because the ears are in communication with the kidney, that the kidney meridian needs to be tackled directly, for instance.

A good acupuncturist is going to need a lot of time at the first consultation in order to make a thorough analysis of the patient. Every human being is unique and has his or her own constitution. That's why the acupuncturist listens to the patient's entire story first. Only then does he start with a thorough analysis before starting a series of jabs.

With acupuncture, one usually works directly with needles, but there are other possibilities, such as:

- **Electroacupuncture** typically involves an electronic device that stimulates the acupuncture points, though it is also possible that a voltage is passed through an inserted needle. Electroacupuncture has the advantage of delivering constant stimulation while requiring no manipulation by the acupuncturist.

- **Laser-acupuncture** features a thin laser beam that stimulates acupuncture points, rather than a needle.

- **Moxa-acupuncture** consists of warming up the acupuncture points with a moxa stick, which looks like a fat cigar and is made of mugwort herb (Artemisia Vulgaris). These glowing cigars can also be used to heat up inserted acupuncture needles.

- **Cupping-acupuncture** is a method in which a glass bulb is placed on an acupuncture point until it is sucked dry.

- **Acupressure** does not use needles. Instead, the thumb or index finger is used to place intense pressure on acupuncture points. This method is less effective than the acupuncture needle, but since this can be performed at home, I will go into further detail below.

- **Ear Acupuncture** Our entire body is projected onto our ears. The nervous system, circulatory system, muscles, bones, limbs, as well as the endocrine system and internal organs are like tiny projection points available for Acupuncture. In a normal healthy state, we never feel any pain in our ear when pressure is exerted. If there are problem areas, they will be stimulated with needles, electricity, heating, magnetic rods or massages to heal the corresponding body parts. If needles are used, then using the term ear acupuncture is accurate; otherwise, you're likely talking about auriculotherapy.

4.2   Acupressure

In acupressure use is made of:

- Traditional acupuncture with its 12 main meridians and two auxiliary meridians.

- Muscle meridians that run through tendons, muscles and joints, and are energetically connected to the main meridians.

In acupressure one exerts very powerful pressure on an acupuncture point with the thumb or forefinger. I say very powerful pressure deliberately, because initially the pressure must be unpleasant; otherwise pressure must be increased. This unpleasant feeling in the beginning soon disappears and is followed by a feeling of numbness or tingling. The direction of the finger pressure massage is critical. This is because a meridian system has a directed flow. Each point is massaged for a few minutes in a circular motion, preferably in the specified direction or in clockwise direction in which an intense, slightly painful, anaesthetizing feeling arises. Especially in the case of chronic tinnitus, a minimum of twenty treatments are necessary to achieve results.

Since tinnitus is a very difficult disease to treat, I'll give you some (acupuncture) points you can use yourself, or rather, that someone else can use to help you. Note that the direction of the pressure massage is very important. Try not to let the pain get to you in the beginning because I can assure you that this discomfort will eventually disappear.

For stimulation of ear points, blunt objects like matches or fingers are best. It is also very important to move the thumbnail around for a while in order to find the sensitive point. Finding certain points can be a difficult task. Of course, right ear tinnitus should be treated in the right ear and vice versa.

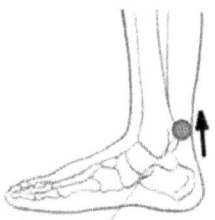

Between the inside of the ankle bone and achilles tendon (pulse perseptible).

At the base of your neck on each side simultaneously. Ask a friend to press inward and down at 45°.

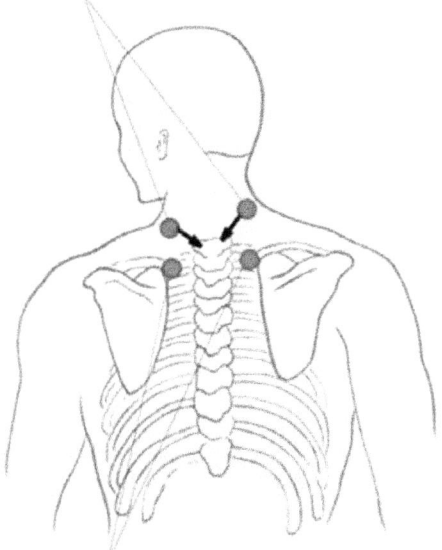

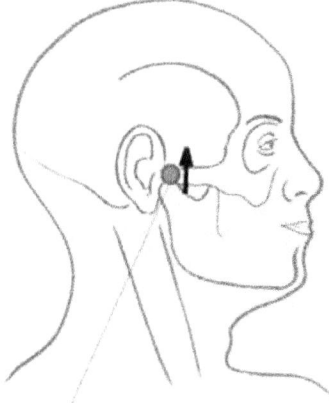

Located against the hinge of each jawbone, touching the front of the ear.
Open lightly your mounth.

On the superior aspect of each scapula or shoulderblade, where the second rib passes under.

At the points where the breast muscle joints the breastbone or sternum.

On the outside between red and white flesh

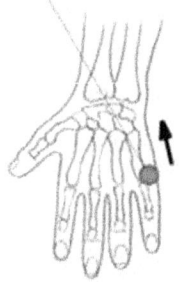

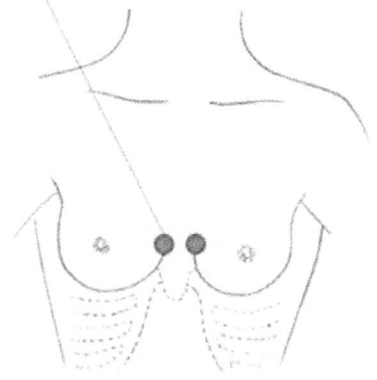

There are some variations of acupressure, namely Shen Tao Shiatsu, Jin Shen and Do-in. They are all based on finger pressure.

4.3 Tai-chi

Tai chi is a relaxing martial art that uses flowing movements to develop the body and mind. A beneficial daily practice that promotes health, Tai Chi is known for its relaxing effects. Furthermore, Tai Chi promotes the lymphatic system, increases oxygen intake and calorie burning, and purifies the body of harmful substances and bacteria.

The three primary components of Tai Chi are meditation, movement and breathing. The floating movements soothe tired and irritated nerves and remove tension from the muscles.

The main form is the short yang form of 37 movements. Although it is a short form, lasting only about 10 minutes, it takes time to get the hang of this. Most beginners take one to two years to master the short form fully.

4.4 Qigong

Qigong (or chi gung) means "working with energy." Specifically, qigong, which originated in China, is the art of using energy to promote health and vitality. It involves the ancient Chinese kinematics that help combat stress, prevent many types of diseases and promote fitness and relaxation. Chi is the energy of life, the vital force in all living things, the life force of the body and mind.

Qigong consists of exercises that keep the chi of the body up to the proper standard and flowing throughout the body. There are many varieties of qigong that all incorporate different movements; essentially, they consist of two groups. The first group includes exercises in which the body is brought into a certain position and then remains static. These silent exercises usually involve meditation. The second group consists of dynamic exercises which are executed slowly, evenly and elegantly. These require relaxed muscle control. With qigong exercises, you will learn to control the flow of chi and send generated energy to places in the body that need it; in this case, the ears and brains. Practicing qigong means re-educating your mind and body. Through the graceful exercises, you will learn a new way of life that will lessen depression, stress and fatigue, and will make your life richer and more enjoyable.

4.5 Foot reflexology

Foot reflexology, or reflexology, embraces foot massage on one hand, and a form of acupressure on specific points of the foot on the other. Reflexology assumes that all our body parts flow into reflex points located on the bottom of our feet via power lines. By stimulating a reflex point via point massage or pressure, the corresponding organ is affected. When a pain point is found, pressure is increased until this becomes extremely uncomfortable. The pain soon subsides, however, resulting in a positive reaction in the corresponding organ, which in our case is the ears. Massaging these reflex points stimulates energy throughout the zone and thus clears blockages in the corresponding organ. When putting pressure on a sore point, one pulverizes and distributes crystals (smaller than grains of sugar) that are beaten down in the zone. It is assumed that these crystals create blockages and congestion in the circulation of the body, disturbing the corresponding organ. When these crystals are crushed and eliminated, energy can return into the flow zone unhindered. When examining tinnitus with reflexology, it is important to include the liver and kidneys.

4.6 Ayurveda

Ayurveda is a Sanskrit word meaning "the science of life and longevity." Ayurvedic medicine is based on classical Indian medicine, the ancient wisdom of health and healing. The method aims to both maintain good health and cure disease. Ayurveda considers health to be a perfect balance between the three fundamental energies of the body called doshas: spe vata, pitta and kapha. They depart from the universal energies (air, fire, water, ether and earth), combining these five elements to the three fundamental energies, the doshas.

This holistic practice incorporates nutrition and diet, lifestyle, exercise, rest and relaxation, meditation, breathing exercises, and medicinal herbs. In addition, Ayurveda includes cleaning and purification programs that heal the body, mind and soul.

According to Ayurveda, tinnitus is a vata disorder. Vata is the energy of movement. Vata regulates all activities in the body, both mental and physical. Vata is therefore responsible for our breathing, the beating of our heart, and all movements in the cytoplasm and cell membranes. Essentially, vata regulates all our impulses in the kilometers-long network of our nervous system. If this vata energy is out of balance, anxiety, nervousness, cramps and tinnitus results.

Here are instructions you can use to alleviate tinnitus, according to Ayurvedic medicine:

- Make a tea of equal amounts of chamomile, cinnamon and comfrey. Use1 teaspoon of this mixture per cup, 2 to 3 times a day.

- Take 200mg Yogaraj Guggulu with hot water 2 to 3 times a day after dinner. Yogaraj Guggulu is a blend of Ayurvedic herbs that soothes Vata and strengthens weakened nerves.

- Rub the teat bone behind the ear with warm sesame oil. Try this for at least a week in the morning and evening.

- Put a few drops of garlic oil at room temperature, in the diseased ear at bedtime. Garlic oil is made by heating sesame oil with minced garlic. Heat the oil, putting pressure on the garlic regularly so the medicinal properties of garlic are easily absorbed by the oil. Once the garlic turns brown, remove the pan from the heat and let it cool.

- Use Ayurvedic Hinjawadi, or Apamarga oil to treat your tinnitus.

4.7 Yoga

Yoga comes from Sanskrit and means "union" or "bringing together." It came into existence more than 4,000 years ago in India. Originally, yoga meant to achieve a deeper state of meditation. In the West, yoga only began to become well-known in the last half of the twentieth century. This usually doesn't revolve around meditation, but rather relaxation exercises that are perceived as beneficial. Yoga to us, called hatha yoga, consists mostly of physical postures and breathing techniques.

Yoga not only provides inner evolution on an energetic level, but also on a physical level. It makes your body stronger and healthier. Different postures activate muscles that we hardly use in everyday life. Yoga stretches the muscles that store tension and brings the body back into balance. By focusing on poses and controlling breathing, we eliminate energy blockages and get a pleasant tingling sensation; this means our energy is circulating again. We feel back in harmony, both mentally and physically.

There are many other types of yoga that have evolved over time, including:

- **Power yoga** that concentrates on the physical strength, stamina and balance.

- **Chakra yoga**, a spiritual approach to the energy fields in the body.

- **Tantra yoga**, which is based on mystical spells.

- **Mantra yoga,** based on mystic sayings and vibrations, called mantras.

- **Kundalini yoga** that generates psychical power in order to achieve salvation.

- There are a dozen other types of yoga that I will not go into here: Bodhi yoga, dao yin yoga, kriya yoga, Sahaja yoga, Sweda yoga, Okido yoga and more.

Yoga's recent surge in popularity is largely a result of the stressful and hectic age in which we live, as provides an outlet to unwind and relax. People doing yoga for the first time, regardless of their age, soon find that most classical yoga exercises are relatively easy to carry out. Yoga ensures that your mind achieves balance and that you experience less emotional pressure.

4.8 Hyperbaric oxygen therapy

Tinnitus can also find its cause in a shortage of oxygen in the cells. By breathing pure oxygen under high pressure, cells receive enough oxygen to carry out their duties up until the smallest blood vessels. This treatment is carried out in a pressurized cabin where one can treat 6 to 8 patients at the same time. After taking a seat in such a cabin, and after hermetically closing the door, pressure is slowly increased to a maximum of 2.4 bar. Participants then put on a mask and breathe pure medicinal oxygen for half an hour, after which pressure slowly returns to a normal value over a period of 15 minutes. Such a trip lasts about an hour and should be repeated every day for ten days.

Note: hyperbaric oxygen therapy is a very effective form of treatment for acute tinnitus, though slightly less so if the tinnitus is already chronic.

4.9 Hematogenous oxidation therapy

In this treatment, an amount of blood is collected. This blood is saturated with oxygen and irradiated with UV light in a special device. The oxygenated blood is then injected intravenously into the patient. By mixing the collected blood with oxygen and ozone, the cellular respiration and, consequently, the energy supply is improved. Multiple treatments are needed before any improvement occurs.

4.10 Intravenous oxygen therapy

During this dubious and difficult form of oxygen therapy, oxygen is injected directly into the veins.

.

5   RESONANCE THERAPY

Everything, including our bodies, consists of energy (or vibrations). Resonance therapy has been derived from several scientists who assume that every cell in our body has a natural resonance frequency (vibration), which acts as a receiver and transmitter. For various reasons these frequencies can get out of balance, causing sickness.

Below, I give a brief summary of the techniques some scientists use for resonance therapy.

5.1   George Lakhovsky

George Lakhovsky constructed a device (the Multi Wave Oscillator) that made it possible to generate a large field of frequencies. He did this in partnership with Nikola Tesla (who harnessed the power of alternating current and created the induction motor). This device consisted of a large antenna and resonance rings. During treatment, patients lie between these rings, creating an electromagnetic field that is transmitted through the body to relax the body and alleviate depression.

5.2   Royal Raymond Rife

Royal Raymond Rife developed the Molecular Oscillation Resonant Instrument (the MORI). This unit sents subtle flow rates through the body, causing viruses to be destroyed and waste to be removed. The main objective of this painless treatment is repairing damaged organs and tissues. In the case of tinnitus the selected frequencies are: 20, 728, 784, 880 and 2720 Hz.

5.3 Dr. Hulda Regehr Clark

Dr. Hulda Regehr Clark claimed that all diseases are caused by microorganisms and pollution, i.e. parasites and toxins. She diagnosed patients by using a syncrometer (which in practice is not easy to learn). In terms of healing, her method was simple and easy.

According to Clark, the parasite streptococcus pneumoniae is the cause of tinnitus. This parasite can occur in the chronic state after pneumonia or what seems to be a head cold and is always present with an ear infection. The streptococcus often hides in cavities under inflamed wisdom teeth and in the liver. A liver cleansing is therefore very advisable.

According to Clark, there are two methods that can be used to eradicate parasites.
The first involves a mixture of three herbs: cloves, walnut hull and wormwood (artemisia). During the second method, the parasite is eliminated by means of a device, the zapper, which removes parasites with impulses of about 5 volts. In fact, the zapper uses a simple square wave generator of about 32 kHz, so that the harmonics reach a broad frequency spectrum. Since the streptococcus has a frequency of 368 kHz, a direct approach with a function generator on that frequency is much more productive.

5.4 Dr. Reinhold Voll

Dr. Reinhold Voll used Chinese acupuncture points for to determine his diagnosis. The Electro Acupuncture according to Voll (EAV) is a rod that measures the electrical resistance of the acupuncture points on the ends of fingers and toes, where the meridians begin and end. These points are related to certain underlying organs. Test ampoules determine both the cause and the proper treatment for the disease. It's a matter of finding the right medication (usually homeopathic), the exact potency (dilution) and the appropriate dose. The result is a medicament comprised of a substance that has an unique frequency, say an energetic charge, which restores balanced to the diseased body.

6 Sound & Music

6.1 Auditory de-stimulation therapy

In this therapy, also called notched music therapy, patients listen to their favorite music after energies within that music that have the same frequency of the patient's tinnitus tones have been removed. In other words, tinnitus is removed. The intention is that tinnitus-causing neurons do not receive a signal while playing the edited music, thus causing no extra charge. Patients' own tinnitus frequencies make the music complete.

6.2 Masking

During this treatment, tinnitus is masked by different sounds. Such a sound could come from a radio or television, or a fan or air conditioner. Furthermore, there are devices on the market that lend masking a helping hand:

- **Hearing aid:** For a majority of patients, tinnitus is associated with hearing impairment. Through the use of a hearing aid, sounds are amplified so that the tinnitus is pushed to the background. Modern hearing aids come in all designs and colors (and of course in a whole spectrum of prices). Due to microelectronics, they have become as small as ear plugs.

- **Tinnitus masker:** This device looks like a hearing aid but produces its own noise. This noise can be adjusted by the user.

- **Masking device:** This device can produce various sounds, such as running water, rushing wind, rippling brook, murmur of the sea, bird sounds or rain. The disturbing ringing in the ears is not completely suppressed as a result, but becomes easier to tolerate when sounds in the environment or muted music can be heard.

- **Tinnitus instrument**: This is actually a hearing aid with a built-in noise generator. Thus, it is essentially a combination of the previous two devices. Tinnitus is camouflaged by an adjustable noise on the one hand and a strengthening of the ambient noise on the other. Critical to this unit is the so called time lag effect, that is, the absence of tinnitus after switching off the device. This time period should last as long as possible, potentially even until the tinnitus disappears completely. This technique requires a excellent cooperation between the patient, the doctors and the acoustic experts as the frequencies and volume of this instrument require regular adjustments.

- Nowadays there are even apps available for smartphones, iPad and tablets. Usually these apps identify the frequency of your tinnitus, then remove that frequency from your music.

6.3 Sound therapy

It is well known that sound therapy can enhance both performance and mental relaxation. Music in the waiting room provides a relaxing feeling. Music in stores heightens sales and music in factories has been modified to increase levels of production. In the gym you train at the rhythm of the music to take your performance to a higher level. This is why people with tinnitus should listen to music every day. Classical music is preferred. The many high tones, especially violin concertos, give a relaxing feeling, make tinnitus bearable and train the brain.

6.4 Sound enrichment

Finding a quiet area, or crawling into a cocoon-like place, is devastating for someone with tinnitus. In a quiet environment, tinnitus is too noticeable. Therefore it is better to have natural ambient sounds. Noise from the radio, television, traffic or recorded nature sounds will more or less suppress tinnitus. There are even special sound pillows with built-in speakers that others will not be able to hear.

6.5 Sound healing

Sound healing is a powerful energetic medium that penetrates deep into the body and mind. Sound massages provide physical relaxation, well-being, growth in consciousness and rest. Singing bowl music in particular is a means to creative atmosphere focusing on security, peace and trust. Sound therapy that employs eg bowls is an energy relaxation method that affects the physical and mental state through the hearing and brain. The use of overtones, music and nature sounds is a boon for the harmonious life energy, vitality and a greater listening, and concentration ability, especially for people with tinnitus.

7 Psyche & Spirit

For curing or reducing tinnitus the use of medications, diet and alternative therapies alone is never enough. The mind of the patient is critical as well. His tinnitus makes him unable to live freely and be at peace with himself and his surroundings. For this reason, psychotherapy becomes the next step.

7.1 Tinnitus Retraining Therapy (TRT)

Learning to deal with symptoms and learning to reverse the negative feelings caused by tinnitus is difficult.

TRT rehabilitation is based on a model described by Jastreboff that shows that tinnitus becomes a problem when it evokes an emotional response. Such a response makes the brain increasingly active, bringing tinnitus to the forefront more and more frequently. As tinnitus sounds increase, so does the emotional response. To break this vicious circle, one can undergo the TRT treatment, which consists of two main parts.

The first involves direct information on tinnitus in general. The aim is to interrupt the negative thought process and make the patient conscious of the fact that it is possible to live with tinnitus. The second part makes use of sound enrichment via a noise masker. This device must be used at least 6 hours per day. The aim is to change the perception of one's own tinnitus such that it fades into the background more and more.

Unfortunately, TRT is being cited as a sort of panacea too often. TRT provides some improvement, especially for hyperacusis, but does not contribute to the recovery.

7.2 Autogenic training

Autogenic training is a form of concentrated relaxation. One learns to tighten his own muscles and relax. As a result, one can relax the muscles and raise the body temperature in certain places through suggestion and concentration. Body control is achieved in steps by attaining a healthy body mind and spirit through both the conscious and subconscious. The first step is learning to control the body and the activities that are generally not subject to the will. During the subsequent steps, one practices various aspects of feelings of the limbs and then switches to the development feelings of the body. Upon reaching the highest level, it is possible to ask questions to the subconscious mind and to receive response. The whole exercise is designed to give people the opportunity to control their body and soul.

7.3 Cognitive behavioral therapy

Cognitive behavioral therapy was originally developed for the treatment of anxiety and depression, but has also been used successfully for the treatment of tinnitus. It is believed that a certain event or situation does not cause emotions, but rather the way in which this event or situation is observed. The primary goal of this therapy is to change the way people think about tinnitus and its effects. It comes down to seeing processes of perception and emotion in a new light to improve quality of life and well-being.

7.4 Regression therapy

The primary purpose of regression therapy is to understand the negative events that became triggers for tinnitus. Under therapeutic guidance, past traumatic events are re-lived. Once they are overcome, tinnitus symptoms no longer have a root cause and may disappear.

.

7.5 Hypnosis

For this treatment to be successful, it is first necessary that the patient is willing to undergo hypnosis and is open to the process. In hypnosis, the psyche is affected under a special form of suggestion. The process of suggestion works to partly disable consciousness until a patient ceases to wholly respond to stimuli from the outside world yet remains extremely sensitive to words he hears. At this point, when the patient hears spoke words, he becomes convinced of his healing.

7.6 Sanjeevini healing

Sanathana Sai Sanjeevini are healing vibrations of spiritual healing. Sanjeevini symbolizes the eternal knowledge of liberation on a spiritual level. Sanatana is Sanskrit for "timeless." In each of us the Sanatana veils energy causes of all healing. Awakening this divine energy (Shakthi) enables real healing to take place. Everything has its own unique frequency, from people, plants and animals to rocks. Unnatural disturbances such as radiation, stress and an unhealthy diet, bring unwanted frequencies into the body, causing an imbalance. By aligning our own vibrational frequencies purposefully one uses different Sanjeevini cards. These cards are divided into two groups: 60 symbols that focus on certain body parts and functions and 186 symbols directed at symptoms and imbalance. This workbook is easy to print online so this therapy, which one performs himself, is completely free of charge.

7.7 Support group

A support group is an important source of social and emotional support. Such an environment enables people to avoid isolation and loneliness and find recognition and acknowledgment. A support group helps participants come to terms with themselves and their situation, and make the best out of challenge circumstances. A support group can organize people in similar circumstances, in the form of meetings, chat rooms, forums and similar platforms. This way, they are able to make a positive contribution to the health of their peers while receiving information specifically designed to meet their needs via leaflets, brochures, books and magazines. Due to a lack of understanding from friends and relatives, people with tinnitus often come to stand alone. Joining a support group gives them a new circle of friends, social contacts, security and familiarity. A self help group is capable of helping participants emerge from a deep valley and get back on track to achieve a state of physical, mental and social well-being outside of the group.

.

8 Smells & Colors

8.1 Aromatherapy

Aromatherapy uses essential oils from aromatic plants. Aromatherapy, or the aromatic medicine, does not make use of scents, but rather of aromatic substances obtained from plants. These aromatics, or essential oils, contain many activating components that can treat various physical symptoms.

In the case of tinnitus, the following oils can be used:

- Pomerans tree; Citrus aurantium or bitter orange tree (has a very pleasant smell). Effective against doggedness, anxiety and nervousness.

- Straw Flower; Helichrysum italicum (very expensive oil, but works quickly and effectively)

- Dragon; Artemisia dracunculus. Dragon Oil provides psychological resistance and combats mental weakness. It strengthens the immune system and stimulates the circulation.

Use 2-3 drops (diluted emulsion of 5-10%) in the ear canal 3x a day. Caution: do not drop directly into ears, but rub a few drops around the beginning of the ear canal with your fingers.

Important notes:
- Essential oils must never be put in the ear in their pure form. They always have to be diluted with a vegetable oil, up to about 5%. This corresponds with 1 drop of essential oil in 20 drops of vegetable oil. For the vegetable oil, you should use cold-pressed wheat germ oil, jojoba oil, sweet almond oil, sesame oil, pure liquid coconut oil or hazelnut oil. I

highly recommend that you drop the first few drops onto your skin to make sure you are not allergic or hypersensitive to the emulsion.

- The aforementioned oils (with the exception of almond oil) are not recommended for use during pregnancy.

The following remedies can also be very effective for the treatment of tinnitus. Take one or more of the following five oils:

- Juniper (Juniperus communis) is an invigorating steam distillate that provides energy and combats fear and weakness.

- Cypress (Cupressus sempervirens): This essence belongs to the mineral onyx (see minerals). Cipresoil works like a pat on the shoulder; it reinforces a disrupted nervous system and brings it back into shape.

- Lavender (Lavandula officinalis): Lavender oil is mainly used to treat sleep disorders, nervousness, stress, depression, anxiety and irritability. This oil primarily brings balance.

- Birch (Betula lenta) is a dry distillation that purifies the blood, and supports wound healing It has a pleasant fragrance and is ideal for the treatment of muscular pains.

- Straw Flower (Helichrysum italicum) is a very expensive oil, but has a tremendous healing ability. It serves as a tonic for the nerves, enhances positivity, and supports a healthy emotional processes in humans.

Make this into a 10% dilution using a neutral carrier oil. Rub 3-4 drops near the front and rear of the ear(s), as well as the back of the neck, 2-3 times a day. This remedy stimulates your blood circulation, supports the nervous system, improves lymph drainage and helps relax the body. Note: this is not ideal for use during the first three months of pregnancy and is not suitable for children under 12 years of age.

- Mix a teaspoon of base oil with 3 drops of peppermint. Massage this behind the ear(s) several times a day.

8.2 Light & color therapy

Light, or in other words, the full electromagnetic spectrum, ensures that our eye can observe various colors and shapes, in addition to light and darkness. The impact that stimuli we receive through our eyes from light and color has on our being as whole should not be underestimated.

Parallel to the images that we receive with our two eyes is a third view energetic track that pulses to the hypothalamus, via the pituitary gland, to end up in the pineal gland. Our pineal gland contains two types of cells, one of which responds to differences in the lightness levels, and the other to various wavelengths of light, the colors. This is why we perceive the color red as stimulating and blue as calming. Moreover, light is also converted into impulses and sent to the pineal gland through our skin.

Light has an extremely significant effect on the human organism. On a bright, sunny day, we are happier than we are on a gloomy, rainy day. The seasons change our mood and energy. We are most active in the summer; in the winter we sleep and eat more. This is precisely why color serves as a very effective psychological device that can be used to gain access to our emotions and our problems. Our built-in biorhythms correspond to nature in terms of light and color and regulates our blood pressure, heart rate, body temperature and hormone levels.

The current light therapy lamps that are in use either approach daylight (full spectrum) or radiate one specific color. Light therapy has a beneficial effect on our nervous system, our psyche and our mood. Light therapy affects our hormonal system, strengthens our immune system and stimulates the blood circulation in the body.

.

During color therapy treatment, light of a particular color is aimed at a patient who is lying down. Usually this occurs in combination with a massage. Generally, natural colors have a positive effect on patients, while modern, intense colors have a negative effect.

- **Red** works well for anemia, low blood pressure and fatigue. Red is connected to our physical and emotional needs. It gives us energy, passion and desire.

- **Orange** helps relax muscle spasms and dispels fear and phobia. Orange enhances creativity, motivation and joy.

- **Yellow** supports the liver and promotes bile secretion. It is an expressive color that makes us happy and optimistic. Yellow inspires us to overcome obstacles and emotional blockages.

- **Green** calms, reassures and normalizes blood pressure. Pale green is ideal for high blood pressure, while deep green is excellent for low blood pressure. However, hard green and bright green should never be used. Light green gives us a great feeling of expectation, it gives us a clear head without any negative thoughts. Dark green on the other hand brings peace and harmony in our lives. It is the color of healing, hope, kindness and faith.

- **Blue** is a containing and calming color. Blue makes our negative thoughts drift away and makes us calm and pensive. Blue gives us peace, tranquility, self-confidence and more. Blue lowers blood pressure as oxygen increases white blood cell count. Soft blue is a perfect color for the treatment of tinnitus. It stimulates our feelings and pulls us out of a humdrum state.

.

9 Refined therapies

9.1 Homeopathy

Homeopathy was created by the German physician Samuel Hahnemann (1755-1843). He discovered the similarity principle; the homeopathic healing principle *Similia similibus curentur,* meaning "similar things take care of similar things." Homeopathy uses natural products in a highly diluted form (called potency). Hahnemann found that the effect of a drug became powerful as it was further diluted and shaken. Homeopathy, a holistic form of medicine, has the advantage of being a flexible healing method that can be performed by both laymen and medical specialists.

With chronic conditions like tinnitus, identifying one or several helpful homeopathic remedies may be difficult as a homeopathic practitioner must consult a patient initially. A good homeopath studies the patient as a whole to discover the disease that has caused the imbalance. This helps to isolate the underlying sickness factors.

Nevertheless, below I've provided some homeopathic remedies that help against tinnitus in general:

- **Aurum metallicum D6:** (prepared from gold powder); Take 2 tablets 3x a day. Especially for use in case of hypertension, depression or pain.

- **R-29 Teridon-Gastreu:** (Dr. Reckeweg); a combination of Argentum nitricum D30, Cocculus D30, Conium D30 and Theridion curassavicum D30; Start with 10-15 drops 3x a day. After a few days, reduce this to once in the morning and once in the evening. After significant improvement (4-6 weeks), only take once a day.

- **Tabacum D12:** 5-10 drops, 3x daily .

- **Chamomilla:** has a wide range of potencies. Low from D3 to D6, medium from D12 - D30. D3 and D6 can be repeated every 2 to 3 hours until pain lessens. Use medium potencies every 3 to 4 hours, with a maximum of 9 doses.

- **Salicylic acid 6C:** for tinnitus with a roaring noise and hearing loss. Take this 3 times daily for at least 2 weeks.

- **China 6C:** for whooshing or hissing due to disruption to the local circulation.

- **Lachesis D12:** 2x daily five grains.

- **Arnica D30:** a muscle tonic that has merit for the deaf with a buzzing sound in the ears. Take once a week.

- **Cimicifuga D30:** works well if tinnitus is accompanied by tense neck and back muscles. Take once a week.

- **Ferrum picronitrium D30:** Take once a week.

- **Helleborus niger D12:** once a day in case of unbearable drone and noise in the head, accompanied by deafness, forgetfulness and muscle weakness. I personally found this homeopathic remedy to have great results. Ten minutes after ingestion my tinnitus increased, but a few hours later it dropped back below the normal level.

- **Pimpinella D1 to D6**

- **Menyanthes D1 to D3:** 3-5 drops more times a day, particularly suitable for tinnitus in elderly people.

- **Calcarea carbonica;** proves its usefulness if there is hearing loss. Works well with crackling sound as tinnitus.

- **Calcarea Fluorica:** (D12)

- **Iris Versicolor.**

- **Formica Rufa.**

- **Silicea** (D12): with humming noise and old age impaired hearing.

- **Primla Veris:** for buzzing sound.

- **Aethusa:** for whooshing sound.

- **Manganum Aceticum:** for whistling sound.

- **Graphites:** for the deaf with a hissing or clicking sound associated with constipation.

- **Belladonna:** for echoing sound.

- **Carbo vegetabilis:** with ringing noise and in liaison with flu states.

- **Chinchona officinalis:** also named China (see above).

- **Chinium Sulphuricum:** for buzzing and ringing.

- **Kali carbonicum.**

- **Coffea Cruda:** for buzzing sound in the back of the head and for sleepless nights.

- **Lycopodium:** for patients with hearing loss and an echoing sound.

- **Carboneum Sulphuratum**

- **Natrium saliculicum:** not only for tinnitus and hearing loss, but also advisable with Meniere's disease.

The advantage of homeopathic medicines is that they generally have no side effects. It seems logical to me to first experiment with this before switching to traditional drugs. Even better is to first consult a licensed homeopath, who has not only more experience but could form an image of your constitution to ultimately decide which agent and which potency (dilution) is most suitable for you.

9.2 Alfred Vogel

Alfred Vogel (1902-1996) was a Swiss and a pioneer in the world of natural health, though he was not a physician. He was mainly concerned with the relationship between nutrition, lifestyle, constitution and disease. He primarily made use of herbal medicine with medicinal plants from all over the world, especially in the form of ointments, tinctures and homeopathic preparations.

For tinnitus, he had the following natural remedies:

- **Geriaforce.** 15-20 drops 3 times daily or 2 tablets (in case of poor circulation).

- **Causticum D4.** 3x daily 5-10 drops (especially in weakness and complaints on the right side.

- **Cocculus D4.** 3x daily 5-10 drops (especially with dizziness and pain in back of the head).

- **Secale cornutum D4.** 3x daily 10 drops.

9.3 Mineral Therapy (the cell salts of Dr. Schüssler)

Dr. Schüssler was originally a homeopathic physician, but also took a critical view of homeopathy. He was disturbed by the ever-increasing amount of homeopathic medicines, which increasingly were administered in mixed forms (complexes). He focused exclusively on the treatment of diseases by means of biochemical salts. Eventually, he used only 11 minerals in homeopathic form and biochemical ointments.

- Below the Schüssler therapy used in tinnitus:

- Calcium Fluoratum D12 possibly interspersed with Silicea D12. Take 5x1 tablets daily.

- Calcium fluoratum ointment; repeatedly rub behind the ears.

9.4 Bach flowers

Bach remedies, which are extracts of flowers, are intended to affect the personality and negativity of the user's soul.

A total of 38 different Bach remedies exist and are beneficial for anxiety, feelings of inferiority, emotional tension, bitterness, loneliness, melancholy, and more. One must choose the appropriate tool to suit the current state of the patient. A Bach remedy is actually a spiritual healing method that cleanses and strengthens both soul and body using spiritual power. There is also a special recipe on the market called Rescue, which is composed of several Bach resources. This is a first aid agent that can have an excellent effect on someone who is distraught. Rescue can be used long-term and consists of a combination of five flower tinctures, namely Cherry Plum, Clematis, Impatiens, Rock Rose and Star of Bethlehem.

10   Folk medicine

An old folk tale says that rustling noises indicate that someone is speaking poorly about you in your right ear and kindly about you in the left. If you can find out who, the murmuring will end. If only it were that simple.

There are many remedies for which we have our ancestors to thank. Their valuable knowledge and understanding surrounding how to use of local minerals, plants and food medicinally has already been passed down through generations for centuries. Until 1900, people had always been dependent on local foods and herbs. However, with the rise of the pharmaceutical industry, our ancestors' natural remedies fell into oblivion.

 And yet, today there are medicines that are made of 85% traditional plant resources. The global study into the effects of nutrients, plants and herbs has already uncovered many chemical activities that explain why folk medicines do work properly.

The list of natural remedies is endless. This is a good thing, because if one remedy does not help, you can quickly switch to something else. You might have more luck with another type of therapy, and your tinnitus could partially or completely disappear. Most of the solutions I have mentioned in this book are not too expensive and been in use for hundreds, if not thousands, of years. Nothing prevents you from trying more than one solution at a time.

Folk medicine can be a safe and effective alternative to conventional medicine when used properly. This isn't simply because it works, but also because it is practical, easily accessible and inexpensive. Here is a small list of remedies for tinnitus from folk medicine.

You won't have to go to a health store to pick up these remedies; you can easily make them at home.

- Lemon balm: Naturally uplifting and relaxing, lemon balm dispels fear and improves memory, making tea with lemon balm an excellent drink for tinnitus patients. It is a good remedy for headaches, migraines, dizziness and tinnitus. When combined with lime blossom, it helps to reduce high blood pressure.

- Use: 60 gr per 1 liter of boiling water, infuse 10 minutes. Drink 3 cups a day; 1 after every meal.

- Yarrow tea with St. John's wort and rue. Drink 3 cups a day.

- Celandine (Chelidonium majus); popularly known as warts herb. The stem and root produce a thick orange-yellow fluid. This fluid can be diluted with warm water to create tea. One can also use dried herb to make a tea by pouring hot (not boiling) water on it. Drink 2 to 3 cups per day, sipping slowly.

- Immerse the face in a large bowl of lukewarm salt water several times a day.

- Drink carrot juice often; freshly squeezed is preferred.

- Take a chamomile steam bath. Keep the buzzing ear close to the vapor.

- Place a clothespin on the second, third and fourth toes for ten minutes so it pushes down at the bottom well (see reflexology). Also do this in the middle of the index and middle finger (between the second and third phalanx).

- Pour lukewarm saline solution into the ear, then rinse it out after ten minutes.

- Put a few drops of hot basil oil in the ear everyday for 4-5 days.

- A mixture of ghee (clarified butter) and milk. Mix a spoon of ghee in a glass of milk. Drink frequently.

- Grate a clove of garlic with a teaspoon of garlic oil and heat. When this cools down, squeeze the garlic clove dry on your ear.

- Place a few drops of warm sesame oil in the ear (or ears), then after 10 minutes, clean your ear with warm bancha twig tea with a pinch of salt (removes excess ear wax).

- Squeeze an onion and drizzle some onion juice on a small cotton ball. Put the cotton ball in the ear.

- Make Burnet-saxifrage (Pimpinella major) into tea. Drink 2 cups a day.

- Andoorn. Make an infusion of Hedge Woundwort. Put 50 g per 1 liter of boiling water then leave to infuse for 10 minutes. Drink 3 cups a day.

- Meidoorn (Crataegus). Like Andoorn, make an infusion of Hawthorn. Put 50 g per 1 liter of boiling water then leave to infuse for 10 minutes. Drink 3 cups a day.

- Vervain (Verbena). Use 30g of leaves per 1 liter of boiling water. Drink 1 cup after supper.

- Balotte (Ballota nigra). Make an infusion of 50 grams of smelly balotte. Drink 2 cups per day.

- Peach. Make peach or apricot oil by cracking the stones, grinding the kernels and trying to squeeze out the oil. Place 3 drops into the ear(s) every morning.

- Millet. Grate the grains from millet in a pan and mix it with an equal amount of coarse salt (preferably Himalayan Salt). Put this mixture in a bag and place it on the ringing ear.

- Bind a disc of onion behind the ear overnight.

- Swedish herbs. Put a few drops on a piece of cotton wool and place it in the ear. Swedish herbs are a blend of 11 pure natural herbs and ingredients in herbal medicine that have been of great significance for over 100 years. Swedish Herbs are a house patent agent that was compiled at the beginning of the 18th century based on old data.

- Mistletoe (Viscum album). Mistletoe tea is made by letting the herb infuse all night, sifting it in the morning and then warming it up. Mistletoe is an indispensable remedy for circulatory disorders. Everyone should do an annual mistletoe tea cure. Such a cure takes 6 weeks: 3 cups a day for 3 weeks, 2 cups a day for 2 weeks, and finally, 1 cup a day for 1 week.

- Petroleum therapy. A great alternative to more dated folk medicine petroleum remedies is the homeopathic remedy petroleum D4 (I have personally gotten good results using this homeopathic remedy).

- Dry some flowers from a cyclaan and crumble them. Fill a small mesh bag with this powder and put it in the ear(s) overnight.

- Put a warm compress on the neck before bedtime. (This promotes good circulation).

- Place 1-2 drops of fresh onion juice in the ear(s) 3 times a week.

- Chew on extra dried fruit for a prolonged period of time.

- Passionflower: 2 mg reduces stress and increases circulation.

- Vinpocetine, extracted from periwinkle. This derivative improves the flow of oxygen to the brain, and increases the blood flow.

- Feverfew. This also promotes healthy blood flow in and around the brain. It's less expensive than vinpocetine, but is also less effective.

- St. John's Wort. This strengthens the nervous system and can also be useful in repairing damage to nerves of the inner ear.

- Regularly drink tea made from the following seeds: sesame seeds, sunflower seeds and fenugreek seeds.

- Daily foot bath with mustard powder. To improve circulation, put about 30 grams of mustardpowder in 10 liters of 37 ° water and soak feet for at least half an hour. Afterward, wash feet with warm water and massage the pads of your feet. This is where the ears' reflex points lie.

- Pouring water round the ear. First, close the ear off then let a small stream of water circle round the ear. Alternate using warm and cold water. This process improves circulation in the inner ear and strengthens the auditory nerves.

- Make a tincture of small burnet.

- Drink tincture of onion. 2x5 drops per day.

- Anti-Tinnitus Tansy Tea: blessed thistle, caraway seeds, sweet woodruff, valerian root and rue. Drink 3 cups a day.

- Boksdoorn. In Asia, the fruit of the Chinese wolfberry (Lycium) has been used as a remedy for tinnitus for thousands of years. Lycium contain not only many nutrients, but also traces of germanium, which has a well-known reputation as an oxygen transporter and appears to have a restorative effect on genes.

11 Nutrition

By now everyone knows that healthy food, like a nutritious breakfast, is very important. A balanced diet is essential in order to stay healthy and fit. After all, our body needs nutrients to function properly. Healthier foods have become popular and much has been written about them; however, many people are eating without taking time to consider what they like. There is an important connection between what you eat and your tinnitus. Tinnitus can be caused by a chronic problem with the metabolism. Our inner ear is completely dependent on our metabolism (metabolic rate for oxygen), our food (nutrients) and sugars (glucose). A healthy and appropriate diet and lifestyle can dramatically reduce your tinnitus.

A complete vegan diet can even work wonders. A vegan diet consists solely of fresh fruits, vegetables, whole grains and beans. All meat, eggs and lactose products are avoided.
To maintain your metabolism and keep your glucose levels stable, abide by the following rules:

- Lactose products: avoid or limit. Goat milk is preferred to cow milk.

- Avoid processed and packaged foods (as they contain too much fat and salt).

- Don't eat fast food.

- Don't eat canned food.

- Reduce use of salt.

- Reduce refined sugars (cakes, pastries, ice cream, candy). Avoiding refined sugar completely is even better.

- Avoid saturated fats.

- Glutamate (flavor enhancer) is out of the question.

- Drink red wine in moderation. Organic wines contain less sulfites.

- Avoid ripe bananas.

- Limit soya intake.

- Avocados can be detrimental.

- Limit coffee to 2 cups a day.

- Drastically limit alcohol.

- Quinine (as in Tonic) can cause tinnitus.

- Limit certain types of chocolate. (Dark chocolate with reduced sugar is best).

- Avoid fast carbs like white bread and pasta.

- Drink at least 5 glasses of water each day.

- Eat more fruits and vegetables.

- Smoking is out of the question.

Vitamins (from "vita" = life) are not foods in the technical sense of the word, but they should be used to supplement the diet. They should be included in the diet under all circumstances, even in minuscule amounts. Vitamins regulate chemical processes in the body. Both vitamins, minerals and trace elements pick up the energy from the food, strengthen the bones and regulate hormones. Even with just one element missing, the body becomes imbalanced and can no longer function optimally. To make up for this, we use nutritional supplements.

- **Vitamin B12** is a folic acid that plays an important role in the functioning of our metabolism and nervous system. It is essential for cell division and the formation of red blood cells. This supplement should always be taken with folic acid. Take 1 mg daily. Sources of vitamin B12 include oysters, milk and dairy, lamb, eggs, fish and poultry.

- **Vitamin B6** ensures healthy nerves and improves mood for people with depression. Take 50 mg of B6 3x daily. Is found naturally in bananas, fruits, vegetables, whole grain products, milk products and eggs.

- **Vitamin A** is an important vitamin for a healthy eardrum. Vitamin A is particularly useful in the treatment of hearing disorders (such as ringing in the ears) that come with aging. This is primarily found in oily fish, blueberries, carrots, oranges and apricots.

- **Pycnogenol** is an isolated OPC (oligomeric procyanidins) extract made from pine bark, grape seed or peanut shells. Grape seeds are the best source of pycnogenol.

- **Chinese foxglove (Rehmannia glutinosa)** stimulates the kidneys and enables the blood vessels to relax. Take a maximum of 1 spoon of liquid extract or 3x daily 5gr powdered root made into tea.

- **Chinese angelica (Angelica sinensis)** This herb expands the smooth muscles in the arteries so that blood can circulate better through the body. The preferred dosage is 3 capsules of 520 mg 3x daily.

- **Feverfew (Tanacetum parthenium)** is especially useful for people who have both a tinnitus and migraines. The phytochemicals in feverfew prevent thickening or clotting of the blood and provide blood vessel spasms. Take 350 mg three times daily as a fresh leaf tea.

- **Black cohosh (Actaea racemosa, Cimifuga racemosa)**, also called Cimicifuga or lice herb.

- **Vincamine** is periwinkle extract. Vincamine increases the blood flow to the brain, which in turn improves memory and concentration. Usual dosage is 60 mg a day.

- **Vinpocetine** is actually a derivative of vincamine. Keep the dose to 10 mg per day.

- **Spirulina (Arthrospira Platensis)** is a saltwater algae that serves as a complete and nutritious food supplement.

- **Magnesium** is a mineral that is greatly involved in our energy production, muscle relaxation and nerve function. Green vegetables like spinach and turnip leaves are especially rich in magnesium. 400 mg per day is the recommended amount.

- **Zinc** concentration in our inner ear is significantly higher than in the rest of our body. A deficiency can easily cause hearing loss, typically during old age. 30 mg is recommended. Don't exceed 80 mg daily. Zinc can primarily be found in lamb, cereals, eggs, oysters, fish, beans and pumpkin seeds.

- **CoEnzym Q10 (CoQ10)**: 200 to 300mg daily.

- **Piracetam** increases intelligence by replenishing the brain and increasing its activity.

- **Beetroot** is a powerful detoxifier.

- **Iron** can be found in kale and parsley.

- **Folic Acid** can be found in kale, peppers, spinach and beet tops.

- **Chrome**. Apples and green peppers contain lots of chrome. Chromium regulates the metabolism of glucose and protectants against hypoglycemia.

- **Choline**: For example, choline can be consumed via beer yeast daily or 2 lecithin tablets 3x daily with meals. Beans are also rich in choline.

- **Apple cider vinegar** Take 2 tablespoons of honey with 2 spoonfuls of apple cider vinegar daily with a glass of water.

- **Ginkgo**: Ginkgo biloba has a beneficial effect on the circulatory and central nervous system. Ginkgo is primarily used to improve memory during aging.

- **Garlic** prevents clogging of the arteries.

- **Fresh pineapple** contains a high dose of vitamin C, which is a strong antioxidant.

- **A three-day diet of only fruit and vegetable juices.** Purification cures are galore. Because many books have already been written on this subject, I will not dwell on it here. Still, I do recommend that everyone to do a cleansing treatment at least twice a year. Your body and your tinnitus will be improved.

- In the sixth century, the physician Trallianus wrote the following about tinnitus: "Rub cedar rosin vinegar or snails and centipedes in oil behind the ear." I've tried plenty of things to cure my tinnitus (see my story), but I will leave the latter remedy to someone else.

11.1 Enzyme therapy

Enzymes control the chemical processes in our body. They are protein-like substances that act as catalysts. The construction of hormones also depends on enzymes. Enzymes stimulate the regenerative ability of our cells. They normalize the energy production in the nervous system and take care of organ innervation.

In nature, enzymes are primarily formed by the germination of seeds. A healthy diet that includes fresh raw plants, and especially germs, will provide us with the enzymes necessary to prevent many diseases. A shortage of enzymes is the primary cause of arteriosclerosis, nervous disorders, poor circulation and more. There's a very simple solution for this problem: put wheat grains, lentils, mustard seed, flax seed, alfalfa or other organic seeds in lukewarm water in your kitchen and let them germinate. There is no better diet than one made up of germinated seeds.

11.2 Macrobiotics

According to macrobiotics, the primary cause of tinnitus is the intake of sticky and high-fat food. In particular, yogurt, ice cream and other dairy products, as well as sugary sweet foods such as chocolate, sugar and honey are problematic. To reduce, and in most cases, stop the whistling, buzzing and other disturbing noises, use these tips on macrobiotics:

- Eat as many whole grains as you can with every meal. Eat black rice, buckwheat and other black or dark-colored grains in particular.

- Try to avoid flour, polished and refined grains and cereal.

- Eat more beans, especially lentils, black beans, chickpeas and akurdi beans, because they strengthen the ears.

- Regularly eat bean products like tempeh, natto and tofu.
- Limit your intake of juice, salt, animal food (yogurt, ice cream and other dairy products), as well as simple sugars (refined sugar, honey and chocolate).

- Avoid inaudible, low-frequency sounds (motorcycles, cars, airplanes and power transformers). Vibrations of low frequency cause stress to the inner ear.

- Make an equal mix of dried daikon, aduki, kombu and shiitake mushroom. Pour in 5 times as much water and gently bring it to boil for 30 minutes. Take 1 cup a day for 10 days.

- Place a ginger compress around the ears.

- Cover the ear with the palm of your hand and firmly tap it with two fingers of the other hand for 50 to 100 times.

- Reduce intake of all hard baked flour products such as bread, biscuits and cakes.

- Tea from dried daikon is ideal against all ear problems. Dried daikon is stronger than fresh daikon and can be used for a long period. Use 1 part soaked dried daikon in 4 parts water. Bring this to boil and let it simmer for 30 minutes over low heat. Add a pinch of salt in the last 5 minutes. Do not sweeten.

11.3 Food for thought

11.3.1 Dopamine

Dopamine is a neurotransmitter that is responsible for a healthy immune system, a properly functioning nervous system and a healthy assertiveness. Alcohol, nicotine and sugar disturb the dopamine balance and cause an addiction over time. Good food sources for the production of dopamine include eggs, fish, meat, dairy, cheese, nuts and seeds, legumes and avocado.

11.3.2   Acetylcholine

This neurotransmitter is the primary chemical carrier of thought, memory and our ability to concentrate. Choline repairs damaged brain cells and thereby enhances memory. Food in which choline is present in strongly includes: free range eggs, soybeans, lecithin granules, brewer's yeast and whole grains (wheat germ).

11.3.3 GABA (gamma-aminobutyric-acid)

GABA is a calming neurotransmitter. Low GABA levels cause anxiety, irritability and insomnia. Alcohol, benzodiazepines and barbiturates cause a decrease in GABA levels. Positive dietary sources of GABA include seeds, fresh nuts, potatoes, broccoli, green vegetables, free-range eggs, bananas and onions.

11.3.4 Noradrenaline

Norepinephrine is a major excitatory neurotransmitter that we need for concentration, motivation and alertness. It's a "happy-maker," and thus partly responsible for a dynamic and active day. The vitamins B3, B6, C, folic acid, iron, copper and sufficient oxygen increase noradrenaline levels. Food sources are the same as for dopamine.

11.3.5   Serotonin

Serotonin a calming neurotransmitter that is responsible for a normal sleeping pattern, healthy appetite, normal blood pressure, constant body temperature, and a decent working memory. A lack of serotonin is the primary cause of depression, aggression, insomnia and eating disorders. Sugary foods should be avoided at all times. Instead increase the use of brown rice, bananas, sunflower seeds, pumpkin and sesame seeds.

12 My Story

After hearing an intense noise, my right ear suddenly started ringing. Being quite loud, it sounded as though a kettle was constantly being heated on the stove. And I also seemed to become more sensitive to other noises on top of it. In other words, I fell victim to tinnitus and hyperacusis. This was the start of years-worth of misery.

In the beginning, I visited several ENT doctors. The first one ordered a hearing test and prescribed a cortisone treatment (Medrol). This five-day cure relieved me of my tinnitus...for five days. At the next visit, my doctor simply prescribed Sibelium and Dogmatil. Sibelium is a remedy for treating heart disease and high blood pressure; my blood pressure has never been high. Dogmatil is an anti-vertigo product; I had never had vertigo. A second ENT doctor gave me another hearing test and prescribed cinnarizine (again an anti-vertigo drug!). The third ENT doctor again performed a hearing test and also a Bera test.

The results were obviously negative, except for a small dip at 12 kHz in the right ear and minor hearing loss, but this was normal at my age. The doctor's conclusion: the whistle will never go away; you'll have to live with it. He told me that over the years, the whistling will become less of a nuisance, which he claimed to know from experience as he could hear the humming of the fluorescent lights in his practice at times. His decision was like a slap in the face. I felt as if I was terminally ill and didn't know how long I had left.

When I went to the next doctor, I got a referral to a psychotherapist. That's how he got rid of me. Such a consultation should be free. No cure should mean no payment, just like in China. There, you pay the doctor to keep you healthy and you don't have to pay if you're sick. With all due respect to conventional medicine, I think if this system were implemented outside of China, many doctors would go bankrupt.

At that point I'd had enough. Instead of choosing to take my leave of this world, I decided to do anything possible to find a way to silence the kettle. I was obsessed with gaining knowledge about my disease (symptom, actually).

To make a long story short, here's a summary of what I've done over the past years:

- Chiropractic: 5 sessions

- Osteopathy: 5 sessions

- Acupuncture: different acupuncturists. Many therapists have shaken my hand and given me false hope. They all start with three sessions and end up with at least 5 to 10 sessions. Then they kindly explain that there is probably nothing more to do, or they send you to a colleague known for another sort of therapy. Thus, you are sent on a wild goose chase and the years of misery fly past.

- Gallbladder and liver cleansing: Annual (with magnesium sulfate or Epsom salt)

- Cleansing diets: a dozen

- Nutritional supplements: a dime a dozen and I still take them.

- Tinctures: I have had over 100 different homemade ones and I'm still working on drinking all of them.

- Swedish herbs: I walked around with Swedish drops in my ear for 5 weeks. After that, I drank a lot of them.

- Enzymes: to strengthen the adrenal glands.

- Hematogenous oxidation therapy: 5 sessions

- Homeopathy: too much to list.

- Hyperbaric oxygen therapy: 10 sessions. The first ENT doctor I went to turned down my proposal of hyperbaric oxygen therapy. A few years later, I'd gotten so far as getting a doctor to give me a certificate for ten sessions in a diving bell. If I had had those 10 sessions in the first few months, then I would have probably never gotten tinnitus, but then again, this book would also have never been written.

- Tai-Chi: two years of intensive Tai Chi Chuan short version of 37 movements.

- Qigong: 2 years intensive.

- Fitness: several years intensive.

- Foot reflexology: 3 sessions

- Ear candles: I applied a dozen of them after therapy.

- Electroacupuncture: 5 sessions. Have since bought an electrical apparatus so I can overflow several acupuncture points myself regularly.

- Resonance Therapy: Since my profession was electronics, I was already in possession of a function generator, frequency counter and oscilloscope. So for me it was easy to apply the appropriate frequencies related to tinnitus on myself with some homemade brass handles and brass footrests.

- Relaxing music CDs: various

- Books: I've read and bought piles of books, even though each one only contained one remedy for tinnitus.

- Sauna visit: regularly. I have already installed a full-spectrum infrared sauna at home myself.

- Colour Light Therapy: specially purchased and built into my sauna.

- Crystals: I walked around with an onyx crystal in my pocket for years.

- Bach flowers: some therapies.

- Gemmotherapy: especially rowan

- Aromatherapy: various oils.

- Folk Medicines: galore.

- Nutrition: Ever since I got tinnitus, I've attached great importance to a healthy diet. Ready-to-eat products aren't allowed in my house anymore. I have not drank coffee in years. I only drink purely roasted chicory coffee (rightly called the Belgian ginseng). I rarely eat bread, just spelt bread. For breakfast I eat oatmeal. I also try to eat as much gluten-free and sugar-free food as I can.

Sure, I can keep going with this list; but the question is, what has actually helped? In short, everything and nothing. After one year, my hyperacusis was as good as gone. After two years, I was able to drive my car without using earplugs. After four years, my tinnitus was drastically reduced. Most of the time, I simply don't think about it. I've been able to sleep without background music for years now.

The majority of the day I just do not think about it anymore. Only driving the car is risky, especially on the highway. If I were rich, I'd buy a luxury car that doesn't make a lot of noise. A silent electric car would be even better. Perhaps the increasing number of vehicles is not only the biggest polluter, but also the biggest contributor to the increasing number of tinnitus sufferers. Transformers and oscillators increase my tinnitus. I can spend a couple of hours in front of a computer, just like I can watch a couple of hours of television. Previously I could not get closer than 3 feet to a classic TV unit. Those old TVs with a CRT have a heavy oscillator of 15625 Hz for imaging. They are real electro-cannons aimed at the viewer. With the new LED flat screen TVs, I have no problems.

If each remedy I took and each therapy I underwent over the years reduced my tinnitus by 1%, then my tinnitus has been reduced by more than 70%. A healthy diet and appropriate lifestyle helps partially. Homeopathy helps partially. Oxygen therapies helps partially. Acupuncture and acupressure helps partially. While a MAGICAL cure for tinnitus doesn't exist, there are many solutions that suppress those noises in your head, if they don't make them disappear completely.

.

13   Conclusion

If the remedies listed up to this point have not satisfied your wishes, I will comment on the following treatments:

- **Inner warmth meditation:** Visualize heat in the body to relax all your muscles and destroy negative feelings.

- **Salt body scrub**: The intention here is to remove dead skin cells and stimulate blood and lymph circulation.

- **Nod finger method**: Cover both ears with your palms so the fingers point at each other behind your head. Place your index finger over the top of the middle finger and snap them on the underside of the skull. Do this 40-50 times. Repeat this process several times a day until tinnitus reduces.

- **Ear candles** are hollow candles made of linen soaked in beeswax, herbs (such as sage, chamomile, St. John's wort), essential oils and honey extracts. Ear candles are cleansing, giving an intense feeling of pleasant warmth and a pleasurable feeling. The pure beeswax soothes the entire ear. It is assumed that it activates the blood circulation and lymph flow. Note: I'm against using this therapy with a perforated eardrum, epilepsy or an ear infection, because the use of ear candles can also be dangerous.

- **Periostmassage**: This method concerns the periosteum, which is derived from the Greek words "peri" (around) and "osteon" (bone), and refers to the membrane that surrounds bones. The periosteum is composed of an outer layer of connective tissue and an inner layer with nerves, blood and lymph vessels. A rhythmic pressure massage improves blood circulation and metabolism locally.

- **Reich massage**: Coupled with breathing techniques, reich massage works to relax to relax unconsciously tense muscles (because of neuroses, emotions and fears).

- **Vegetotherapy**: This treatment assumes that tinnitus is set in motion by emotional stimuli, which results in tension in the autonomic nervous system. One tries to ease tension through emotional expression.

- **Laser therapy**: Laser light is aimed directly at the eardrum.

- **Magnetic field therapy:** This therapy uses pulsating magnetic fields to facilitate the transport of ions across cell walls. We all know that our body cells vibrate at a certain frequency that varies from organ to organ. Magnetic field therapy attempts to recover damaged nerve tissue by bringing malfunctioning or acidified cells back to proper frequencies.

- **Iridology:** Derived from the Greek words "Iris" (rainbow) and "scopeo" (to look at something), Iridology is an alternative diagnostic method that Chaldeans and Aztecs were already practicing 3,000 years ago. According to this mehtod, by examining the iris of an eye, one comes to know what is going on in the body. All bodily organs are apparently represented in a specific part of the iris and a defect is expressed through a change in color, form, brightness or depth. One can look at the iris with an illuminated magnifier to observe defects. This method is capable of diagnosing both existing health problems and past ones.

- **Mindfulness**: A therapy to experience less stress and get more out of life. On the one hand the base is a form of meditation in which one becomes aware of the physical and mental conditions of the moment. On the other hand mindfulness helps to accept the current attitude. People pay conscious attention to the tinnitus and learn to accept that it is part of their lifestyle.

- **Gemmotherapy**: Gemmo therapeutic extracts are produced by maceration of buttons and / or young shoots. People use the embryonic form of the plant that contains all essential components, such as plant growth hormones, vitamins, trace elements, minerals and the sap of the tree shrub. Rowan is the most appropriate product for tinnitus. 5-15 dr. / Day.

- **Stones**: Healing stones are not inanimate objects, but living beings who, much like humans, plants and animals, emit their own vibration. The ancients knew that gemstones belonged to the natural medicines. They didn't wear them to show off; they carried them with as if they were companions and healers. Cava composite, ammonite and onyx in particular are stones used for people with tinnitus.

- **Applied Kinesiology**: This method is similar to Dr. Voll's electro-acupuncture, but mesures muscle tension instead of acupuncture points.

- **Sublingual drop test**: During this text, one drips cooking oil of a certain type under the tongue. Similar to homeopathy processes, this broth has been diluted multiple times. Two drops are placed under the tongue. A reaction should take place after 20 minutes for cases of tinnitus. Then, placing drops of a more diluted version of the same substance will neutralize the effect of the first drops. A great deal of discussion is going on about the results of this healing method.

- Furthermore, you have the cell therapy, own blood therapy, self-urine therapy, endobionts, neural therapy, nosode therapy and more.

Information and knowledge are often the first steps towards the acceptance and lifestyle change. I hope tinnitus sufferers find a partial, if not complete, solution to their problem by reading this book, and I hope that solution opens the door to a better, happier life.

Just as every color is a mixture of the three main colors, the classic remedies in this book can be combined with homeopathic remedies, essential oils and Tai Chi or something else. Any remedy that may improve your quality of life is worth giving a try.

If one in ten people suffer from tinnitus, then, certainly some of your colleagues are bothered by the same pest. You regularly pass people with tinnitus in the supermarket. In a crowded theater or cinema, there are at least ten cases of tinnitus. Not everyone you see on the street with a hearing aid is hard of hearing; many, albeit reluctantly, wear a masker.

If one in a hundred, or even one in a thousand, tinnitus patients have been helped in part or completely by this book, then I'm happy. In that case, I'm proud to help a couple of people from their misery, from their cocoon, their daily torture so they can build a new life; a life full of peace and relaxation. A life where you can relax in peace and quiet and read a book or even do nothing at all. A healthy life with work, hobbies and friends. I sincerely hope that you will be after reading this book, one of those people.

.

Literature

Behr, V., *Was der Arzt verordnet*, Bruno Wilkens-verleg, Bad Bevensen, 366 p.

Bottigelli, G., *La Farmacia del buon dio*, SM Silvio Mursia, Milano, Italy, 1978, 172 p.

Brian, L., *Tinnitus no more*, 2012.

Carter, M., *Body reflexology*, Prentice Hall, New Jersey, 1987, 216 p.

Coleman, W., *Tinnitus treatment*

Dalet, R., *Supprimez vous-même vos douleurs par simple pression d'un doigt*, Opera Mundi, 1978, 159 p.

Devlieghere, G., Vanhove, M., *Etherische Oliën*, De Eenhoorn, Wielsbeke, 1999, 160 p.

Mann, F., *Genezing door acupunctuur*, De Driehoek, amsterdam, 143 p.

Fischer-Rizzi, S., *Hemelse Geuren*, De Driehoek Amsterdam, 1993, 232 p.

Fröhling, I., Jacoby, B., *Vitalität und Gesundheit durch Licht*, Falken-verlag, Germany, 1998, 96 p.

Hempen, C., H., *Atlas van de acupunctuur*, HB, Baarn, 2008, 304 p.

Houston, F., M., *The healing benefits of acupressure*, Keats Publishing, Connecticut, 1974, 96 p

Huijsen, L.P., *De homeopathie-gids*, Homeovisie, Alkmaar, 1988, 287 p.

Kenyon, J., N., *Acupressure Techniques*, Thorsons Publishers, 1987, 159 p.

Meyer-Camberg, E., *Lexicon der natuurgeneeskunde*, De Driehoek, Amsterdam, 324 P.

Oberbell, K., *Fit durch Vitamine*, Südwest Verlag, München, 1999, 223 p.

Pahlow, M., *Geneeskrachtige kruiden*, Uitg. Helmond, Helmond, 1984, 466 p.

PARKER, D., *Color Decoder*, Quarto Publishing, London, 2001

Péron-Autret, J.,-Y., *101 trucs de medicine naturelle*, Librairie Hachette, Paris, 240 p.

Price, A., *Tinnitus stop*, 2012.

Rannou, A., *Mooi gezond met een appel en een ei*, Bosch & Keuning, Baarn, 1978, 238 p.

Test-aankoop, *Geneesmiddelen Mythes en Feiten*, De verbruikersunie, Brussel, 254 p.

Treben, M., *Gezondheid uit de apotheek van God*, W. Eensthaler, Steyr, 100 p.

Uyldert, M., *Genees U Zelf*, De Driehoek, Amsterdam, 381 p.

Uyldert, M., *Lexicon der Geneeskruiden*, De Driehoek, Amsterdam, 351 p.

Van Baarle, F., *Geneesmiddelleer*, Standaard Wetenschappelijke uitg., Antwerpen, 416 p.

Van Os, F.H.L., *Gids voor geneeskrachtige planten*, Reader's Digest, Amsterdam, 476 p.

Van Stuyvenberg, W., *Vitamines en mineralen*, Elsevier, Amsterdam, 228 p.

Verbeke, G., *Klankschaal-abc*, Empty Sky, 2000, 151 p.

Vogel, A., *Anders beter worden*, Kosmos, Antwerpen, 1990, 616 p.

Vogel, A., *De 100 beste tips*, Mix Media, Harderwijk, 1996, 157 p.

Voorhoeve, J., van Vliet, H., *1000 homeopatische raadgevingen*, La Rivière & Voorhoeve, Kampen, 1989, 203 p.

Wolffers, I., *Medicijnen*, Contact, Amsterdam, 2007, 1006 p.

Woollerton, H., J. McLean, C., *Acupuncture energy in health and disease*, Thorsons Publishers Ltd, Northhamptonshire, 130 p.

Ypma, R., *Aroma- en kleitherapie*, Ankh-Hermes, Deventer, 2005, 96 p.

www.ingramcontent.com/pod-product-compliance
Lightning Source LLC
Chambersburg PA
CBHW070847180526
45168CB00002B/985